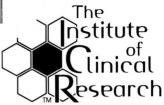

The
Institute
of
Clinical
Research

raising standards
sharing knowledge
developing professionals

The leading organisation for clinical research professionals

Internationally recognised as the premier organisation for clinical research, respected as a key influencer, promoting knowledge and understanding by engaging the healthcare community and the general public.

Raising standards

The Institute's professional standards encourage our members to work to the highest standards, enhancing the standards of clinical research and maintaining the professional identity of members

The Institute recognises the academic achievement and clinical research experience by awarding designatory letters e.g. MICR to our members.

Sharing knowledge

The Institute offers a comprehensive range of Information Services and publications, including our journal Clinical Research focus, our publications, online resources, a resource centre and membership helpline.

Developing professionals

The Institute provides educational courses and training workshops, continuing professional development, academic qualifications and accreditation of training courses. All of these enhance the professional competence of our members.

For more information call +44 1628 899755
or visit www.icr-global.org

About the Author – Martin Robinson

Martin Robinson was educated at The University of Bath, England, where he obtained a PhD in Biochemistry in 1984. He has over 20 years experience in the pharmaceutical/biotechnology industry and has held a variety of posts during his career, covering drug discovery, international clinical study monitoring and clinical trial project management. He has worked in drug development Phases I-IV and has been involved in protocol writing, CRF design, writing patient information leaflets, data management, preparing clinical trial reports and writing SOPs. Martin's therapeutic area experience includes oncology, infectious diseases, depression, hypertension, and HIV.

Martin is employed as a Training Consultant for the ICR. His experience as a trainer spans a decade and involves designing and delivering educational programs for staff involved in clinical drug development. Subjects include clinical study monitoring, personal development courses for CRAs, problem solving and process improvement facilitation, project management training and consultancy. Martin has co-authored a book about risk management in clinical research.

Foreword

Good writing skills are critical for clinical research professionals. The ability to write clearly and concisely is an essential factor not only in communication but also in the creation of the documentation, which makes up a complete and robust audit trail. Nowadays we communicate by writing almost every day. Can you remember the last time you were in work and did not send an e-mail?

The key to successful writing is understanding through clarity. This book will help you keep things simple, avoid misunderstandings and adopt appropriate writing styles to suit the medium you are using. Written language and style evolve with time. One aspect, which remains constant, is the need to provide a clear message. I hope you find this book useful in making writing an enjoyable and fruitful experience for both you and your readers.

Contents

Introduction

Writing is a form of communication and we review how the whole process works from the writer to the reader. We look at occasions when a relatively informal style can be used such as in e-mail. At the other end of the spectrum a more prescribed approach is needed in writing letters, drafting reports and creating SOPs. We examine techniques for writing clear patient information sheets so that they are effective in ensuring clinical trial subjects are informed as part of the consent process. We will see how following a few simple rules can boost the clarity of our message and keep it concise. These guidelines can also reduce some of the grind and feeling of foreboding we sometimes experience when writing. Report writing is covered by looking at issues such as our target audience, report structure, avoiding jargon and finally some tips on writing monitoring visit reports. We review the methods for writing clear and practical SOPs. We will examine some useful techniques in reviewing work so that we look at our own creations through fresh eyes, giving us the ability to spot errors and make improvements. Reviewing other's work and giving feed back is another key skill we will cover. For those of you who are interested in taking writing further, there is a section on writing creatively for journals or you may even have a book in mind.

Chapter One: Writing and the Drive to Communicate

Human beings have been communicating using the written word for thousands of years. The earliest form of a written language seems to have evolved in ancient Mesopotamia (now part of Iraq) 5000-6000 years ago. Scribes used a wedge-shaped stick to press symbols into clay which was then hardened to make a permanent record. This style of writing, known as Cuneiform, was used to make records including a ledger of rented land, monthly accounts and harvest yields. Writing seems to have evolved with the development of agriculture, which created a need to keep permanent records.

The hieroglyphs of ancient Egypt, dating from 3000 BC have been well documented and have allowed us to gain a deep understanding of life in that period across a wide spectrum of Egyptian society. The rise of the Greek and Roman empires gave birth to the modern form of writing we recognise today in the western world. Not only was writing used for letters, legal documents and comprehensive financial records, but also significant literary works were created. These societies produced great scholars and philosophers including Homer, Aristotle and Socrates. It is through the written word that an unbroken chain of learning has been passed down through the ages to continue today as modern day students continue to study classical works such as Homer's 'Iliad' and Aristotle's 'On Youth and Old Age, On Life and Death, On Breathing'.

Since those ancient times mankind has tried constantly to make the written word as widely accessible as possible. The printing press, invented by Johann Gutenberg in c1450, made the mass publication and circulation of literature achievable. Our subsequent ability to produce and distribute books and newspapers in huge numbers contributed to this drive.

Nowadays, due to the combination of widespread literacy and the development of a variety of technologies for recording and distributing information, the written word can be broadcast simultaneously to billions of people across the globe. Recent developments such as e-mail and texting by mobile have accelerated the evolution of written language. The message CU L8TER :) is almost a return to the hieroglyphics of 5000 years ago.

The communication process

The urge to communicate using writing is a major human need. We converse on many levels but the principle is always the same. We communicate for a purpose. It may be to make something happen, to issue a statement of intent, to record a fact, a belief or an event. We can imagine communication as a multi step process. Whether or not we achieve our intended goal depends on how the whole chain of events works. This process of communication is broken down into component parts (Figure1). We can imagine these as the sender of the message, the message content (the words), the medium, the receiver of the message and the ultimate effect of the message – the result.

Figure 1 The process of communication

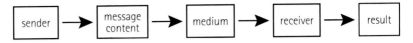

The end result of our communication is dependent on the four preceding steps of the process.

What's in it for the reader?

Successful communication involves managing all parts of the process so that the receiver will act according to our wishes. It is clear that there is plenty of opportunity for the message to get scrambled and the reader to act in a way which is not in keeping with what we had in mind. Maybe they will not act at all and in some cases, may chose to ignore our message entirely, with all the frustration that involves. The secret is to put ourselves in the shoes of the receiver. What's in it for them? How will they perceive the message? Will they understand it?

If we look at the communication process we see that the sender is at the start of the chain. The reader of the message may choose how to act on our message depending on how they regard us. This may include factors such as their perception of our:

- Status

- Level of education

- Company or organisation

- Level of influence over them

- Cultural background

We may have little or no control over these factors particularly if this is our first contact with our intended recipient. We will certainly make an impression on our reader by the way we craft the wording of our message.

A key step is to attract the reader's attention. If we are sending an e-mail or letter then the title needs to reflect the subject of the message. If we are writing a report we must make it concise and easy to read but with enough detail to satisfy the reader's need for knowledge. The reader will make judgements about the importance, formality and urgency of our message based on the wording and how we structure the sentences and paragraphs. If the reader does not know us, these factors will have a powerful influence on the impression they may form about us. We will be looking at these issues in greater detail in subsequent chapters.

The Institute of Clinical Research

The next aspect of the communication process involves the medium. Nowadays the choice is widening in the way we communicate. From one aspect this is extremely helpful. It allows us more flexibility in how quickly and widely we communicate. The drawback is that with more options open to us, there comes the increased risk of making a poor selection. Some issues such as negotiations, giving bad news, and those which require detailed discussion are best handled by face-to-face communication. Documentation may be produced once the face-to-face discussions have taken place to record and confirm what took place and what was agreed. There was a famous case in the UK just after the turn of the 21st century, when a company informed its staff of their impending redundancy. Rather than calling a meeting and then dealing with each employee individually, the company broadcast the news by a text message to the mobile telephones of its staff. Naturally this caused great distress and the story made the national news. TV footage showed groups of upset and angry employees complaining bitterly about how insensitively the company had handled the situation. The employer's point of view was that they had wanted to communicate the information quickly and simultaneously to all employees. While news of redundancy can never be an easy message to communicate, the company was left to reflect on a public relations disaster. In the following chapters we will look at how best to use the various media of written communication and their respective advantages and shortcomings.

The final piece of the communication process is the reader of the message. The background of the reader is one of the most powerful influences in how the written message will be interpreted and acted upon. One way of considering this is to imagine that there is a filter, which is used by the person reading the message. This filter is responsible for how the reader interprets the message. This filter is influenced by the reader's set of values, beliefs, cultural issues, own past experience and language skills. This explains why several people may interpret the same message in a number of different ways. We all have our own unique view of the world and this influences us in the way we interpret information. A dramatic demonstration of this occurred in Iran in the 1980s when the then UN Secretary General, Kurt Waldheim arrived in Tehran to try to broker an agreement between the US and Iran over a hostage crisis. Relations between the two countries had been poor for some time, but had completely disintegrated when the US embassy in Tehran had been taken over by a mob that was holding the US diplomats and their staff hostage. Kurt Waldheim held a press conference on landing at Tehran airport in which he said he was there to 'mediate between the two sides in order to reach a compromise'. Several minutes after leaving the airport on the way to the negotiations Mr Waldheim was shaken and bewildered when an angry crowd gathered and began stoning his motorcade. Apparently the meaning of two key words had got lost in translation. 'Mediate' had been interpreted as 'meddle or interfere' and 'compromise' had been taken to mean 'undermine'.

The past experience of the reader influences how they respond to different types of messages. Most people learn that unsolicited or 'junk' mail is of little value to them. The packaging usually reveals it as junk mail even if the envelope is disguised as 'important information'. The first sentence of the letter is usually enough to send it on its way to the waste bin. Equally a bill is all too easy to recognise and we know from past painful experience that we ignore it at our peril and so it gets our attention.

Writing for a purpose

The key to successful communication is to examine the end result we wish to achieve. Is it to merely update our intended reader with information or is it to persuade them to take a particular course of action? In clinical research there are many occasions when we are documenting the events that took place so as to maintain the integrity of audit trails. But who will study this information and why? We need to think of the end purpose when we are communicating in writing.

It is worth mentioning the occasions when writing is not the most appropriate form of primary communication. Writing should be avoided as a primary medium when:

- Giving bad news

- Complex information needs to be exchanged, to allow immediate questions and clarifications and avoid misunderstandings

- Negotiating

Written communication can be a very powerful medium and we need to consider carefully what we are trying to achieve when using it. If the purpose is to provide information what will the reader do with it? Does the reader actually need the information or just selected parts of it? How much detail is required? What other information does it need to cross-reference? Very often in clinical research, the regulations and guidelines determine the information we need to provide. For example when a Sponsor applies for a clinical trial authorisation, the appropriate documents need to be completed accurately before submission to the regulatory bodies. Complying with regulations often gives little leeway in the type of information required. This can be both a help and a hindrance depending on the scope for interpretation of the questions that need to be completed. It becomes more complicated when we are faced with a blank sheet of paper or computer screen and we need to consider how to craft the message carefully to achieve the desired result.

One way to help this is to consider that communicating using writing has the following general purposes:

The Institute of Clinical Research

- To ask for information
- To provide information
- To record something that took place
- To provide a statement of intent
- To request a particular course of action
- To influence or persuade people to our way of thinking

We will be looking at the various examples above particularly with respect to the clinical research environment.

Chapter Two: You've got mail

Receiving mail, whether it is conventional or electronic, can produce a variety of emotions in us depending on the sender, the appearance of the message and the content. Even before we have opened our mail and studied it we might be filled with feelings of dread (inland revenue, exam results) or keen anticipation when we recognise the writing or e-mail address of a friend we have not heard from for some time. We may choose not to open our mail but to discard it immediately if it looks like unsolicited junk. Sometimes this is the toughest barrier to overcome when we are sending mail to very busy people who may be used to making snap judgements about whether or not to open our message. A particular case comes to mind of a phase IV study where much of the communication was done by the Sponsor using overland post to over 2000 Investigators. The key was to make the envelope look business-like while at the same time giving it an interesting appearance so that the recipient would want to open it – a major challenge!

With the advent of e-mail the emphasis and use of both conventional and electronic mail has changed. Both e-mail and standard mail have their place as key communication tools. We will look to see how they can complement each other and circumstances when one form may have advantages over the other.

Life before e-mail

It is hard to imagine business and social life before e-mail. All written communication sent to a distant receiver was confined to conventional overland mail, telegram or facsimile (fax) transmission. Faxes are faster than overland mail but are more time consuming to send than e-mail. After all, we have to get up from our desks, walk over to a fax machine, dial the number, feed the paper in and so on! Both overland mail, telegrams and fax transmissions suffer from a weakness. The sender of the message will always be in some doubt about whether the intended recipient has received it. Of course a letter can be sent registered mail. However when received in a busy office, any number of people can sign for it and the intended individual recipient may still have been in ignorance of its existence. Fax transmissions are vulnerable to mechanical failure, and sometimes the fax machine at the receiver's end has run out of paper! Only a follow up telephone call from the sender was a sure fire way of discovering that the intended destination of their message had been reached.

With the advent of e-mail came the ability to communicate with vast numbers of people worldwide, simultaneously and at almost real-time speed. As with many inventions the benefits are often obvious. Any drawbacks manifest themselves sooner or later. How often do we bemoan a development that should have made our business lives easier? Common complaints include the amount of e-mail waiting for us when we get back from holiday, being copied on messages unnecessarily, and receiving text that cause us offence. In some instances it may be a case of crocodile tears. Quite naturally we like to feel indispensable, so receiving hundreds of e-mails a day is a bit like a badge of honour. All of those messages need attention even if it is only to be opened to discover that nothing needs to be done.

Perils and pitfalls

It is the very advantages of e-mail of speed, ease of use and coverage of a wide network that have led to some of the problems we encounter. So how can we maximise these benefits and reduce the drawbacks?

The speed of e-mail puts us all under pressure to respond to received messages. The danger is that we may not give ourselves time to reflect on our reply, especially when we receive a message that annoys us. We can all probably recall a time when we have replied immediately to a frustrating e-mail from a work colleague or business acquaintance as if we were returning a salvo of gunfire. Sometimes sending e-mails in anger can elicit an equally hostile response from the receiver and a very destructive 'e-duel' can result. When there are significant differences of opinion or strong disagreements, the best solution is often to pick up the telephone or arrange face-to-face meeting so that a mutually agreeable solution can be reached.

Unnecessary e-mails to colleagues who work in close proximity to us can be an irritant and often it may be preferable to drop in for a quick chat. E-mail can sometimes make us lazy, and besides, the exercise in walking round to our colleague's desk will probably do us good.

Another aspect of the trigger-happy habits, can be a reply which contains careless spelling, grammar or inappropriate information which may have been part of a forwarded message and which we did not intend the recipient to receive. The spelling and grammar may not matter so much to a work colleague we know well but if we are corresponding with someone on less familiar terms perhaps outside our organisation, it can reflect badly on our own standing in that person's eyes. The organisation we represent will hardly have their reputation enhanced as a result of our carelessness. The added subliminal message is that a badly composed e-mail says that we do not respect the receiver enough to give sufficient care to the information we are sending them.

Because of the ease of use of e-mail it is sometimes very tempting to send too much information in one message. From the recipient's point of view it can be very frustrating to have to keep scrolling up and down the computer screen in an attempt to digest a significant body of work in an e-mail. Choice of font is important too. Some of the more decorative and colourful ones are more appropriate for party invitations than business correspondence. The font size should be big enough so the recipient can read it in comfort but not so large that it gives the impression we are sending an 'electronic shout'. Upper case should be avoided. The receiver's perception may be that we do not respect their ability to comprehend or filter out the key points of our message. Many people find reading upper case more difficult than sentence case. Ironically, text in upper case may receive less attention rather than more.

Who we copy on our e-mails needs careful consideration. We need to ask ourselves why should a particular person receive a copy of an e-mail. Some users will overcompensate and copy a lengthy list of recipients unnecessarily. This can be irritating for some of the people on the copy list who may not understand the reason for receiving the message in their already crowded in-box. If there is no good reason why we should send a message to a particular recipient then we probably should not send it.

Unfortunately we cannot escape office politics and all organisations suffer from this to some extent. Demonstrating our perceived authority by copying in a comprehensive list of who we consider powerful allies often serves only to alienate the intended target of our message. Of course there are occasions when copying a member of senior management (e.g. for information or a status update) is necessary but this should be done with discretion and only when required. E-mail systems are not intended for use as political tools or as threatening weapons.

Our choice of words should convey courtesy, clarity and objectivity. Emotive and accusatory language is to be avoided. We need to think particularly carefully when writing to people for whom English is not their first language. Avoiding colloquialisms, jargon and slang is always helpful. When receiving a message from a non-native English speaker we may need to make plenty of allowances for style and content. Sometimes a message may appear very abrupt or even rude. This may be due to a number of factors including local national e-mail etiquette, expertise in English and cultural issues. English is said to be a language containing more words than any other. Perhaps English people need all these options to express themselves because of their alleged reputation for diplomacy! Many other languages, particularly those from northern Europe, contain far fewer words than English and so there may be only one way to express a concept or idea. This may sometimes appear overly blunt and direct at first glance to a native English speaker, so making some allowances is a good policy.

One aspect of using e-mail as a form of communication, particularly in the clinical research environment, is the lack of robustness in the context of the audit trail. This is due to the ability if the receiver of the mail being able to easily alter the content of the message before printing off a hard copy and deleting the original text. Doubt may be shed on the identity of the sender if security is lax, passwords are shared and PCs and laptops are left unattended and unprotected by screensavers for lengthy periods. A foolproof validated e-mail system which is internationally recognised and use is still some way off at the start of the 21st century. For these reasons e-mail can be considered to be no more than a form of electronic conversation and only hard documents with original signatures have any significant standing in legal, contractual and regulatory issues.

The Institute of Clinical Research

E-mail etiquette and effectiveness

One of the attractions of e-mail can be its brevity and lower level of formality. However, there are still some general rules of etiquette which have evolved.

Some people may choose to address familiar work colleagues with the salutation ' Hi Brian, Amy...' and use a more chatty style to convey the message. Depending on our relationship with our correspondent we may choose to use the more formal 'Dear...' as the salutation and sign off (known as the subscription) with the expression 'Kind/warm/best regards' followed by our first name. It is common practice to add the 'business signature' which may include full name, title, job role, and contact details such as telephone and fax number. Other additions after the signature may include a standard paragraph which contains information as to what to do if the e-mail has been received in error, confidentiality issues and disclaimers.

Consideration for the receiver should always be uppermost in our minds. The message should be polite, courteous and expressed as objectively as possible especially if dealing with an emotive issue. Sometimes a 'cooling off ' period (overnight for instance) is useful before replying to a contentiously worded e-mail and can help us stay calm and objective when we reply. Brevity is also helpful, as is bulleting key points where appropriate and making it clear how we would like the recipient to act on the message. FYI (for your information) is always a helpful cue in the first line of the message. If we need a reply then we should make that clear together with an expectation of the date by when we need it. ASAP is not a particularly constructive or considerate request as what may be possible by our criteria may be undoable from the receiver's perspective and vice versa. Message titles should be given careful thought and need to be brief and accurately reflect the content of the message. When forwarding messages a quick check on the content will ensure that unnecessary or sensitive information is not passed on inadvertently.

If a lot of detailed information is to be sent, it is good practice to include it as an attachment, for example a Word document. Another feature is that the formatting is retained in an attachment document whereas it may be lost when the receiver opens detailed information contained in the body of an e-mail. This makes it particularly difficult to read and the receiver may have to invest some time in copying and pasting the message into a more user-friendly format.

Good etiquette is to ensure the e-mail is spelled correctly as it shows consideration for the receiver. Most e-mail systems have a spell checker so there is little excuse for a poorly spelled message. Of course spell-checkers don't pick up on words such as names, so it's appropriate to ensure you have spelled someone's name correctly or indeed used their right name!

Letter writing – 'snail mail'

Letters on paper still carry great significance as a form of communication despite or perhaps because of the advent of e-mail. Much importance is often attached to receiving a document personally addressed that we can touch feel and personally possess. Various flourishes can be used such as the quality of the paper, the company heading on the top of the page and the pleasing appearance of the document. These factors all point to the amount of time and trouble that has been spent by the sender. Although conventional letter writing is a slower form of communication than e-mail, hence the expression 'snail mail', the power of a letter is undiminished.

In the context of clinical research, correspondence by letter forms a key part of the audit trail. A letter written by a CRA to an Investigator following a monitoring visit, summarising any key findings (both positive and negative) and actions required, is vital in maintaining communication links and clarifying what needs to be done.

Writing business letters

Conventions in business letter writing are more formal and rigid compared to those used in e-mail. The letter needs to include the addresses of both sender and receiver, the date of writing, a formal salutation (Dear...) the subject of the letter as a bold heading (e.g. Re Ethics Committee Meeting Dates), the subscription (Yours faithfully/sincerely), the full name and job role (e.g. Project Manager, Study Coordinator etc.) and the signature of the writer. The address of the sender is nearly always accommodated by the use of pre-printed company notepaper. The name and address of the recipient may need to include their department, especially if they are employed by a large organisation. Nowadays the salutation is nearly always followed by the addressee's name rather than by 'Sir' or 'Madam'. Whether first names are used will depend on the familiarity between the sender and the receiver. If using the more formal approach it is important to get right the addressee's title be it Mr/Mrs/Ms/Dr/Prof.

Including the subject of the letter in bold after the salutation is extremely useful for the reader. It helps them make a quick assessment about the importance and urgency of the content of the letter. Not having to read the entire content of the letter immediately helps a busy person manage their time and will always be appreciated.

The appearance and layout of the letter is very important. There should be a balance between the area taken up by the main text of the letter and the size of the paper. For a one page letter the aim should be to get the text roughly equidistant from the top and bottom of the paper. The margins should be equally proportioned. For a multi-page letter the spacing may need to be carefully adjusted so that the last few words do not run onto the last page. If possible, arranging the text so that a new page starts with a new paragraph is also good practice. The appearance of the letter should be pleasing to the eye and the content easy to read and understand so that the intended recipient is 'invited' to read it.

As with e-mails the style should be concise with the main points listed in a logical order and bulleted if that helps with clarity. The same rules apply with respect to courtesy and avoiding accusatory or emotive language.

Chapter Three: Writing information for clinical trial subjects

The two purposes of Good Clinical Practice (GCP) are to protect the rights and welfare of clinical trial subjects and to ensure that the data generated by a clinical trial are valid. One of the key concepts is upholding subjects' rights and welfare and this is covered in the principle of informed consent.

We know that as part of the informed consent process, clinical trial subjects must be given written information about the trial. The wording must be both comprehensive and understandable. This is to ensure that all relevant details about the trial are given to the subject and that anyone considering participating in a trial understands fully what is involved. Most of us are familiar with the need to use non-technical jargon. The ICH GCP guidelines (reference 1) make this clear in section 4.8.6 which says 'The language used in the oral and written information about the trial, including the written informed consent form, should be as non-technical as practical...' There is still plenty we can do to make it as easy as possible for potential trial subjects to make an informed decision about whether or not to take part.

The paradox: inclusiveness v minimalism

Writing information for clinical trial subjects which includes all the required elements (according to ICH GCP there are 20) while keeping the document concise is a major challenge.

The golden rule is to keep things simple. This does not mean having to use words that only a four year old would understand or patronising our readers in other ways. The concept is to make the work quicker and easier for us to write and more straightforward for our audience to read and understand. At the same time we must make sure our grammar is generally sound and our choice of words and sentence structure carefully considered.

One of the solutions is to keep the number of words to a minimum. There are various methods for doing this. The first is to use active language rather than passive.

Sentences usually have three major parts:

• An agent: the person or thing doing the action

• A verb: the action

• An object: the person or thing that the action is done to

Writing actively involves using these parts in the order of agent, verb and action. A sentence written passively will have the object first, then the verb and finally the agent. To demonstrate how passive writing can be more cluttered and unclear we can look at the following example.

"The nurse will weigh you once a month." This is an active sentence with the nurse as the agent, weigh as the verb and you as the object. Written passively it becomes 'You will be weighed once a month by the nurse'. The active sentence contains eight words, and the passive ten. Using the active form in this simple sentence has reduced the number of words by 20%.

A second technique for preventing clutter is to avoid using 'fillers'. These include words such as 'thus', 'however', 'then' 'also', 'basically'.

'The nurse will weigh you once a month and you will then also need to give a small blood sample. However, every three months your lung capacity will be measured." By removing the clutter these two sentences become:

'The nurse will weigh you once a month and you will need to give a small blood sample. Every three months your lung capacity will be measured.'

Taking out these words also has the subtle effect of appearing to make participating in the trial less arduous for the patient

A third technique is to avoid using cumbersome phrases when one word will do.

'...in order that the doctor can measure your progress'. can be changed to '.....so that the doctor can measure your progress'.

Other examples are included in this table.

Preferred	Avoid
If	In the event of
	In the likelihood of
partly	to some degree/extent
much	a good/great deal of
many	a great many
now/currently	at the present time
most	the great majority
because	due to the fact that
start	embark on
by	by means of
using	

As well as reducing the number of words we can make our work more readable by using plain English. This does not mean using childish expressions or phrases. It involves using straightforward words rather than some of the more long-winded ones that seem to have crept into our language. The result is a crisper, cleaner style, which the reader should find easier to manage. Some examples are shown in the table below.

The
Institute
of
Clinical
Research

Worth avoiding if possible	Simple alternative
utilise	use
deploy	
employ	
exploit	
facilitate	help
additional	extra
supplementary	
terminate	end
commence	start
viable	possible
feasible	
achievable	
consequently	so
permit (v)	let (v)
purchase (v)	buy
endeavour (v)	try (v)
meet with	meet
genuine	real
authentic	
valid	
bona fide	

Sentence structure

As well as trying to keep words to a minimum we can make things easier by making our sentences simple. Long complex sentences are sometimes difficult to follow and some may need re-reading to get the intended meaning. Most people find the ideal sentence length to be around an average of 15-20 words.

Imagine this was a sentence from a patient information sheet.

'At a screening visit you will give your complete medical history, have a physical examination, an assessment for the determination of the severity of your arthritis, pulse and blood pressure measurements will also be taken, and any current medicine you are taking for your arthritis will be stopped immediately, or over the next several days'.

This sentence is 55 words long. It contains several pieces of detailed information covering a range of themes. Broken up into shorter pieces and cutting out some unnecessary words, the passage may look like this.

'At the screening visit you will give your complete medical history and have a physical examination. Your pulse, blood pressure and the severity of your arthritis will be measured. At this visit, any medicine you are taking for your arthritis will be stopped. This may be immediate, or will occur over the course of several days.'

Now the largest sentence length is 14 words and we have used four sentences. We have separated the concepts of physical examination, measurement of disease, and the stopping of current treatment. This should let the reader digest the information more easily and make it more memorable.

Varying sentence length is another tactic we can use to encourage our reader. Here is an example:

'Your doctor has established that you have rheumatoid arthritis. You are invited to take part in a study to look at the effect of Artheez, an investigational new drug to treat your condition. This study involves research.'

The last sentence of four words has the effect of emphasising the research aspect of the study. And it gives the text some 'punch'.

Magic bullets

Another way of presenting information in a readable style is to use bullet points. This is useful if there are several pieces of information we need to include in the same phrase or sentence.

Take the following example:

'Previous research studies in the past and other tests have shown that taking Artheez results in side effects such as mild and infrequent headaches, occasional dizziness, a metallic taste in the mouth, sleep disturbance (rare) and occasionally loss of appetite. '

We can make this more digestible for the reader by using bullets.

'Previous research studies have shown that taking Artheez results in side effects such as:

- mild and infrequent headaches

- occasional dizziness

- a metallic taste in the mouth

- sleep disturbance (rare)

- loss of appetite (occasional) '

Maybe we won't get many patients taking part in this study after all!

Like any technique in writing, using bullet points can be overdone. There is a danger that our document can end up looking like a shopping list, so good judgement is needed.

The most important aspect of informed consent is that the potential clinical trial subjects are fully informed about all relevant features of the trial. The written information is only part of this process. The discussion with the Investigator and their colleagues is also vital and other media may be used, including videos. The written document can be helpful as a basis for the potential subject to discuss issues with their relatives and friends. It can act as a catalyst for questions from the subject. Anything we can do to make it user friendly and readable by adopting the principles we have discussed in this chapter can only enhance patients' rights and welfare in clinical research.

Chapter Four: Writing reports

Reports are written for a range of different reasons in clinical research. We may have been asked to make a recommendation to senior management. Status reports are used by project managers to inform stakeholders of the progress of the study. Monitoring visit reports are required by ICH GCP after each visit by a Clinical Research Association (CRA) to an Investigator site. Both Sponsors and Investigators may be required to write various reports for the regulatory authorities and the Sponsors have to ensure that clinical trial reports are produced at the end of a trial.

Whatever the purpose of a report, the writer will nearly always know more about the subject than the reader. Reports should be clear, simple and easy to follow. As with writing information for patients, the same rules of using plain English apply to reports.

Who's my target?

As with any form of writing, the questions we need to ask are who is going to receive this information and what are they going to do with it. We may be writing a report for a single person, perhaps a committee, or for a range of individual people or groups who each may have different needs. Perhaps we need several versions of the same document, which might vary in detail and length depending on our intended audience. Generally when we write a report we know more about the subject than the reader. We need to make a special effort in getting our intended message across. This will allow our reader to extract the relevant information and take the appropriate course of action.

Our report may be used for providing information such a status update. In this case our report may be circulated regularly to the same group of people who rely on it to be kept abreast of progress, perhaps of a clinical trial project. These people are usually the project stakeholders.

Clinical trial reports have many interested parties including the clinical trial Sponsor, the Investigators (or at least the chief or principal ones), and the regulatory authorities. Each will have a different need for information and so will concentrate on those aspects of the report relevant to them.

Clinical trial reports are often a team effort with contributions from staff from clinical operations, statistics, regulatory affairs, medical affairs and so on. Because everyone has their own style and may be working in remote locations from each other, a Medical Writer coordinates the entire effort. This person ensures that the report conforms to the required format, that it is indexed and the different sections cross-reference each other properly. The spelling must be consistent and error-free, and the Medical Writer checks that the report contains all the relevant sections and information.

Sometimes our report might be for senior management. They may have asked us to research a particular business area and need a course of action recommended. Senior managers usually prefer reports to be kept brief and concise. They are receiving information from various areas of the business or organisation and can be easily swamped with too much detail. On the other hand we do not want to be so brief as to deny them vital information. Picking out what is relevant is the trick. The general rule when judging the right amount of detail is that the higher up the hierarchy the less is needed. This inverse proportion assumes that the higher up managers are in an organisation, the more strategic their role, and hence the need for less detail. A senior manager may need information about the status of 30 projects. If a 40 page report for each arrived on his or her desk each month, our poor manager would soon be drowning in paper. Really valuable and vital information can be communicated in tables, graphs and figures. Appropriate detail can be added to highlight significant aspects such as milestones achieved, issues slowing progress and remedial actions taken. If managers need more detail they can always ask you for it.

Stakeholder	Information required	Level of detail	Frequency
Senior Management	Project status Problems and proposed solutions/ action taken and result	Low level of detail/summary information	Quarterly
Immediate Manager	Project status Problems and proposed solutions/ or action taken and result	Medium level of detail	Monthly
Project Team Members	Project status Problems and proposed solutions discussed	High level of detail	Every 1 - 2 weeks
Suppliers	Specific with respect to supplier	High level of detail	As needed

Structuring reports

Status reports are usually produced regularly, perhaps at the same time in each month. The format of status reports is often pre-determined perhaps by company or organisation procedures. We may have little input into its design. On the other hand, we may have complete control over this aspect. We need to make the report easy for our reader to find their way around and to retrieve information effortlessly. A large report may need a contents page.

The Institute of Clinical Research

Most reports have the following general structures. So if you don't have to follow a particular format this is usually the default to use.

General Structure of reports

Title
This should be kept brief and reflect accurately the subject of the report. In other words 'it does what it says on the can'.

(Executive) summary
This should be no more than one page. This allows someone to quickly get the salient points of the report in no more than about 5 minutes reading.

The purpose of the report
This is a description of what the report is intended to achieve and the terms of reference (if any) under which it was commissioned. This section will present the background to the report and who asked for it and why. This will help you write the report, and the reader to make sense of it.

The methods used to compile the report
This section should explain how you went about collecting the information for the report. You may have had to conduct some research and will need to describe how the data was collected. For example you may have interviewed people or asked for questionnaires to be completed, retrieved information from websites or used reference books. Many of your readers may not look at this section, as the findings of the report may be of more interest to them. However, if this is not routine work and you have had to go to significant effort to conduct the research, you will need to be able to back up your findings and hence your conclusions by showing you have used reliable sources and sound methods.

The main body of the report
This is the detail which contains the findings, reasoning and any arguments. The information should be presented in a logical order to help the reader navigate through it.

The order might be:

1. past
2. present
3. future

or :

1. problem
2. possible solutions
3. options
4. recommendations

Jumbled information is of no help to the reader and much of the value of good work can be lost in a poorly structured report. If your purpose has been to persuade or recommend you will have an uphill struggle if this part is not well written.

The conclusions

This is the part that many of your readers will turn to after they have read the executive summary and is the most important feature of the report. This section should be kept brief and concise. The methods and main body of the report are the foundations on which the conclusions are based. This piece should contain a summary of your findings and recommendations, if any. The conclusions need to be concise and punchy so that the reader is in no doubt about the outcome of the report. Beware of putting new information in here, which is not in either the main body or the methods sections. If you find that happens, review the main body of the report for a suitable place to put the information. Your conclusions should be based on the data presented in the main body. This allows you to keep your arguments concise and to the point.

Appendices

You may wish to add further information, which may not be directly related to the purpose or findings. The idea of appendices is to support the material you have put in the report. The appendices may include a detailed account of the methods you used and other supporting material, or actual reference documents. These are often validations of the methods you have used to compile the information. Including appendices helps avoid distracting the reader with extra material in the main body of the text. This will probably be the part of the report your readers will look at least. Nevertheless it is important as this information supports your methods and findings.

Writing lengthy reports can seem quite daunting. Knowing where and how to start can be a difficult hurdle to jump. One method is to use a technique called mind mapping. This involves using the brain to collect and link related pieces of information. Using this method helps break down the information into manageable pieces. We will discuss mind mapping and its use in greater detail in Chapter 7 when we look at writing articles for journals.

Starting with an outline is another way of marshalling your ideas. In this method you use a blank sheet of paper to write down all your ideas as quickly as you can in note form, letting your thoughts flow. This is sometimes known as 'brain dumping'. Once you have your ideas down on paper you then organise them under headings into appropriate sections and paragraphs using a PC to cut and paste. Of course you may not get all your ideas down in one session. It is a good idea to leave it for a coupe of days and then come back to your outline. You will see it through fresh eyes and more ideas and thoughts may occur to you. You may also change your mind about how you have initially organised your material.

Writing reports so that they are read

As with other forms of written communication we have discussed so far in this book, reports should be written with the reader in mind. We need to make it easy for them to find the relevant information and to be able to easily digest it. We may like to believe that everyone will be interested enough to read every word of our report. Only part of the report will interest most people. Each person may have their own specific interests so 'something for everyone' is generally the reality rather than 'everything for everyone'. This can be handled by sending all interested parties the executive summary and then supplying the detailed report upon request.

Some reports can be quite lengthy. We can help the reader by breaking down the information into smaller chunks. Appropriately titled paragraphs are enormously helpful. The usual rule is to use one concept or idea per paragraph. This allows the reader to skip sections which they may not feel are immediately relevant to them and to concentrate on the issues which they find interesting. In each section or paragraph, start with the most important issues, then follow with the next important and so on. You can go into further levels of detail as the paragraph progresses so that the reader can stop and move onto the next section once he or she feels that they have enough information.

A technique called signposting is also valuable. This involves using side headings and subheadings. These should be used consistently depending on the weight the writer wants to give them. A hierarchy of font size is usually the method of choice, the main headings being in larger type than the subheadings. You may want to number points sequentially. The most convenient way of doing this is to use a system where a single number denotes a main section, a double number a sub-section and a triple number a sub-sub section. An example may look like this:

7   The Need for Standard Operating Procedures (SOPs)

7.1 SOPs are required to help employees follow procedures consistently and correctly. This has been apparent as:

7.1.1 quality standards have...

7.1.2 there have been inconsistencies in...

7.2 SOPs are also necessary for our organisation to comply with regulatory requirements...

7.2.1 Regulations require our organisation to have a quality management...

7.2.2 Regulations and guidelines are not sufficiently detailed to...

Keywords can be emphasised. The most favoured convention is to highlight keywords in bold. This draws your reader's attention to what you want to emphasise.

If your report is to a wide range of people, be careful about using technical language. We have mentioned earlier that the author is often the person who knows most about the subject. Sometimes technical experts fall in to the trap of forgetting that not everyone has their level of expertise. Some even go to the extent of trying to show off the breadth and depth of their specialist subject. Unexplained technical terms and incomprehensible jargon in a report, will put off many readers and much good and valuable work may be ignored or lost. On the other hand, if you are a technical expert you don't want to come across as patronising or condescending. The objective is to get the reader to understand what it is you are trying to communicate. Try to avoid phrases like 'of course', 'obviously' and 'as we can clearly see'. It may be obvious to you, but not so clear to your reader who may have a different perspective. Similarly, your level of interest in a particular aspect of the report may not be the same as your intended audience. If you put in phrases like 'it is fascinating to note' your readers may disagree with you.

Each abbreviation should be defined at its first use. For example, rather than wading into talk about ADRs without explanation, the way to express this would be: 'There were no additional Adverse Drug Reactions (ADRs) to report'. We can then use the abbreviation ADR without having to write it out in full each time. A table of abbreviations is also helpful (as part of the appendices). You may have been asked to write a report for your new manager who has just joined your organisation. They may need help to make sense of the array of abbreviations that will inevitably face them in a new position.

Any figures or graphs should be clearly labelled and accurately referenced in the text. Ideally they should be close to and on the same page as the piece of text that refers to them. This allows your reader to compare your reasoning in the text with the illustration in the figure. It also prevents that annoying need to keep flicking backwards and forwards between pages.

An attractive layout for your report will also make it more readable. The margins should be spaced appropriately left and right, and top and bottom. If possible, avoid breaking sentences and paragraph across pages. This allows the reader to follow your reasoning and line of argument more easily.

Monitoring visit reports: some tips

This chapter on report writing would not be complete without dealing with the subject of monitoring visit reports or site visit reports in general. ICH GCP section 5.18.6 states :

'The monitor should submit a written report to the Sponsor after each trial-site visit or trial related communication'. Each organisation has its own formats and methods for producing these reports. Some basic concepts hold true for all.

Monitoring reports should be concise and to the point. If some aspects of the trial are progressing as planned without mishap, then little needs to be explained for these areas. If problems are occurring, particularly those which undermine patient safety and welfare, or data integrity, then more details are needed. An explanation is required of the issue together with how it is going to be resolved, who is responsible and by when.

Reports should stick to facts and not offer opinions. The monitor may think that the site staff are a bit careless in how they maintain the site file. This is irrelevant and should not be included in the report. What should be detailed are the specific deviations and what the monitor has asked the site staff to do, so that the relevant corrective action can be taken.

Each visit report should be able to exist as a stand-alone document and yet should form part of the continuing story of the progress of the trial at each site. There should be no gaps in information between reports. For example, if the monitor has made the request to have the site file brought up to standard and recorded this in the second visit report, we should expect to see how this was followed up in the third visit report. Without this chain of events linking reports it would be a bit like watching a soap or a thriller serial on TV with key bits of the plot missing from time to time. Continuity in factual visit reports follows the same principles as TV fiction!

Reports are created to provide information. We need to make it as easy as possible for the reader to extract the knowledge so they can make decisions, take action or keep up to date. A properly structured report with the information presented in a logical order and at the right level of detail will get the attention it deserves.

Chapter Five: Writing Standard Operating Procedures

We tend to look on Standard Operating Procedures (SOPs) as a necessary evil and sometimes just evil. However the voice of reason tells us that SOPs are essential for a number of reasons. They help organisations comply with clinical research regulations and guidelines. They give consistency to the way procedures are used and define who is accountable for using them. They set standards of performance and can be useful training tools. They are part of a clinical trial Sponsor's quality assurance and quality control systems as identified in ICH GCP section 5.1.1 :

'The Sponsor is responsible for implementing and maintaining quality assurance and quality control systems with written SOPs to ensure that trials are conducted and data are generated...'

SOPs are becoming more widely required and used in clinical research. Many Investigator sites, or the organisations which employ them, are writing and using them. Ethics committees are introducing and implementing them.

If SOPs are essential why is it that they are sometimes not followed? There may be several reasons for this.

- They are impractical and do not reflect reality

- They may be difficult to access by the users because of the need to control numbers of hard copies

- There are too many of them

- They are not kept up to date with organisational or regulatory changes

- They may be badly written from a number of aspects
    - There is too much or too little detail
    - They contain conflicting information
    - They contain confusing information
    - They are not written in the logical order of the procedure
    - They may be hard for non-native English speakers to follow.

This chapter looks at the important contribution that writing skills can make to an SOP system rather than the mechanics of how SOPs are used in a quality assurance framework. Writing SOPs is not just a box-ticking paper exercise. The documents have to be practical, simple to use and therefore easy to read and understand.

As we have seen before in this book, getting started on any writing project is often the hardest part. None more so than with SOPS. Where do we begin if we are starting from scratch? The first step is to break down partial processes or functions into key areas. If we were writing all the SOPs from a

Sponsor's point of view, perhaps we would map out a typical clinical trial in its component stages. Some examples might be 'Writing the Protocol', 'Designing the Case Report Form' and 'Preparing the Informed Consent Form'. From an Investigator site's point of view, we might map out the journey a clinical trial subject makes from when they are considered for inclusion into the study to when they are followed up after their participation has ended. We must not forget to write an SOP on the set up and the maintenance of an SOP system – an SOP on SOPs!

Writing SOPs – the process

Writing SOPs can seem an arduous task. If we have a process to follow which we can use for each SOP, this can take a lot of the grind away. It also helps to write SOPs consistently and relatively quickly. We can build up quite a momentum once the first few are written as we get 'into the swing of it'. Once we have an initial list of the procedures the following process can be used.

1. Define each SOP's purpose

2. Give the SOP a title

3. Define the scope of the SOP

4. Create a process flow of the SOP

5. Write down the process flow as text

6. Allocate responsibility for each step in the process

7. Add any further information to clarify any steps in the process

Let us have a look at each step in more detail.

1. Define the SOP's purpose

Each SOP must have a distinct purpose and this first step is to define what our SOP is intended to do. This must be a clear short statement. If it is hard to articulate this then perhaps we might not need the SOP. The alternative is that we may need to think about developing more than one SOP to satisfy the purpose statement.

Let us suppose we were writing an SOP on providing written information for potential clinical trial subjects to read as part of the informed consent process. Our purpose statement might read: 'The purpose of this SOP is to produce written information for clinical trial subjects that they understand and which complies with the current GCP regulations, guidelines and data protection laws. Provision of this written information forms part of the process of informed consent to participate in a clinical research study'. You will notice this purpose statement contains quality standards; the need for the subject to understand and the requirement to conform with the regulations. These standards help ensure that the SOP fulfils its intended purpose.

2. Give the SOP a title

Now that we have defined the purpose of the SOP we can give it a title. It is easier to do it this way round. If we cannot define the purpose of an SOP then its title is irrelevant. (Many novels start out this way without a title but with a story line planned. Only when the author has made more progress does the title become apparent!).

The title should reflect accurately what the SOP contains and be written prominently on the cover page. The title is the first reference point the user of the SOP has to make sure that they have identified the right SOP. It is important that the title contains sufficient information about the SOP's contents. The title should be short and contain descriptive action words. If we take the example we are following, the title may read something like 'Creating a written patient information sheet for clinical trial subjects.'

(As well as the title the SOP will have the other usual identifiers such as number, version number, date of release, date when it takes effect, etc.)

3. Define the scope of the SOP

The scope statement of the SOP defines the area of work covered by the SOP and which departments or functions it is relevant to. It is sometimes helpful for the statement to include tasks or areas of work which are not covered by the SOP. Generally the scope statement is written by describing what is covered between the first step in the procedure and the last. For the SOP we are using as a case study, the first step in the SOP might be to obtain a copy of the final clinical trial protocol. (We cannot write the information until we know what is going to happen to each patient according to the protocol.) The final step might be obtaining Ethics Committee approval for the completeness and adequacy of the written information. We cannot use the written information unless it has been granted this approval. However the scope of this SOP does not extend to obtaining informed consent of a clinical trial subject. That would be handled by another SOP.

In this example our scope statement would read. 'The scope of this SOP begins with obtaining a copy of the final clinical trial protocol and ends with obtaining the necessary Ethics Committee approval for the written information.' And we might add: 'The scope of this SOP does not extend to obtaining informed consent from a clinical trial subject.'

4. Create the process flow of the SOP

Now that we have defined the scope of the SOP we have the start and end of the procedure. Creating the process flow involves filling in the bits in the middle. If the users of the SOP have not been involved before in the process they certainly need to be for this part.

The users should create the process flow of the procedure as they carry it out in reality. This is a good opportunity for them to make improvements or refinements, or perhaps agree a consistent procedure. The process can be mapped out on a wall with 'stickies'. This team effort is visual and allows different opinions to be heard. Many SOPs will be able to be mapped out in a linear flow, which is ideal when trying to keep things as straightforward as possible. Some branch points may be needed but keeping the procedure simple is the objective. If you find that you have more than about 15 steps in your SOP this may make it unwieldy to use. An SOP with too many steps will become difficult for the users to read and remember. You may need to rethink the level of detail in describing each step, perhaps combining some of them. Maybe splitting the SOP into two separate ones is the solution. As a rough guide each step needs to be described as a single action verb and to have a single deliverable or output. This allows measurement of compliance when the SOP comes to be used in practice.

The process flow can be retained as a flow chart as part of the SOP. This is easy to reference for the reader and to visualise the whole process on one page.

5. Write down the process flow as text

Once the process flow has been agreed it needs to be written down. One of the users may be the best person to do this. The language should be active, simple, concise and have a mandatory quality to it. An example might be 'Ensure that the written information contains all the required elements according to ICH GCP 4.8.10'. Our single action verb is 'ensure' and our deliverable is a written information sheet containing the required elements. Avoid words and expressions like 'could', 'should' and 'if at all possible' in the procedural statements. These words give the reader the impression that they may use their discretion or implies that there are other options when there are not. Vagueness is also unhelpful. For instance if we wrote 'Ensure the written information contains all the required elements' without referencing which required elements, the opportunities for non-compliance with the regulations would be great.

6. Allocate responsibility for each step in the process

Whoever is responsible for each step is going to depend largely on the job responsibilities within the organisation. The important point here is that only one person or jobholder should be allocated responsibility for the conduct of each step of the procedure. This avoids confusion as multiple responsibilities may mean that everyone leaves the completion of the task to everyone else.

7. Add any further information to clarify any points in the process

More details can be added to the steps in the procedure to help guide the user. Care is needed not to add unnecessary clutter to the document.

Once these steps have been followed for a couple of SOPs, the writing process tends to get easier. A momentum can be built up and a surprising amount of progress can be made once people get into the 'swing of it'. The relationships between the SOPs are easier to track if the writing process is reasonably concentrated. Maintaining consistency is also easier.

Reviewing SOPs

As we have discussed it is good practice to have the users write the SOPs. They may have different styles of writing and different preferences for level of detail. We need a person to take editorial responsibility for the SOPs so that they are consistent in format style and language. It is often someone from an organisation's quality assurance function who takes on this coordination role. The review process should involve the major stakeholders of each SOP, in other words the people or departments most affected by them. This should include the users of the SOPs. Each reviewer should be clear on the purpose of their review so they are not duplicating the efforts of the SOP coordinator who may have already checked the spelling consistency of terminology, and so on. The main purpose of review is to check for clarity of meaning and completeness of the process. There may be practical aspects caused by the impact on different departments, which need to be brought to the attention of the SOP coordinator. The review process should be swift and the coordinator needs to set the reviewers aggressive but realistic timelines within which to return comments.

The ultimate test of an SOP is how easy it is to use in practice and a couple of real life tests for robustness may have to occur before the final refinements are made. In any case, SOPs have to be reviewed on a regular basis for ease of use, compliance and relevance to internal and external factors such as organisational changes or regulatory updates. Generally, SOPs are reviewed every one or two years but maybe rewritten sooner if they prove to be difficult to use. To avoid SOPs dating quickly, associated documents can be created to which the SOPs refer. These documents can be changed without having to rewrite the SOP. Examples of associated documents can include forms or checklists.

Having an SOP system is more than a paper exercise. SOPs are of little help if they are difficult to read and interpret. They need to be practical tools that can be used easily and complied with. SOPs written in a simple active style can go a long way to achieving this.

Chapter Six: Reviewing written work

Why review?

So far in this book we have looked at creating pieces of written work for a number of different purposes. An important task in completing the work is to review it. It could be said that a piece of work is only half finished until it has been reviewed. This chapter looks at reviewing one's own work and other people's.

Reviewing is an important process because it can detect:

- Errors in facts

- Spelling mistakes (even after using a spell checker!)

- Grammatical errors

- Faulty sentence structure

- Unnecessary words or phrases

- Poor choice of words

- Unnecessary repetition

- Errors in punctuation

- Unclear meanings

- Inconsistencies in style and formatting

Reviewing may also be used to pass judgement on a line of argument or reasoning from a scientific paper, journal article or recommendations from a report.

Reviewing your own work

Reviewing our own work can sometimes make us cringe. It is bit like watching yourself on video. 'Do I really look like that?' becomes 'Did I really write that?' However awkward this feels we need to face it. It is much better to detect your own mistakes first before other people find them for you.

The first step, if you have created a document electronically, is to spell-check it. The spellchecker finds misspellings but not miss-sense. If you have spelled manager as manger this will not be picked up. A clinical trial manger is not the most suitable place to conduct a research study, not on human subjects anyway. Other common undetected words where the intended spelling is wrong are 'trial' and 'trail'. Each clinical trail should have an audit trial, or is it the other way round? If you have a particular weakness in certain words it is a good idea to use the search facility. Searching on 'trail' will pick up all the occasions you have used the word. You can then check to make sure whether it is used in the right context or not.

Short pieces of work, such as letters, can be reviewed quite quickly. Reading the piece aloud to yourself (without disturbing your workmates) will help you pick up any mistakes in sense and expression. Points where you breathe naturally are sometimes a good indication of where to put commas. If you run out of breath before the end of a sentence then some alterations are probably needed to its length. As a good guide, sentences should be no more than 15 - 20 words long.

Some people find reviewing from the printed page easier than from a computer screen. It is easier to spot errors in formatting, margin widths, font type and size on hard copy. For documents of more than two or three pages, creating a hard copy is very worthwhile.

Reading aloud will pick out words or phrases that you may have inadvertently repeated in close proximity to each other. For instance you may have written 'Please would you arrange to have the CRF queries answered before my next visit. I would like to arrange my next visit for ...' The words 'arrange' and 'my next visit' occur very close to each other in consecutive sentences. This is not technically wrong. It just sounds a bit clumsy and untidy. Perhaps a better way of expressing this might be 'Please would you have the CRF queries answered before my next visit. I would like to arrange my next appointment to see you on ...'

For reviewing longer pieces of work such as articles or large reports, the process is more time consuming. Creating these documents often involves more original thought and creativity than the stock expressions used in letters. Sometimes expressing new concepts in writing may need several revisions before we are satisfied with the end result. The danger in reviewing one's own work is that we are 'too close to it'. Larger pieces of original work have usually needed proportionally more energy and time. It is quite natural that we may feel reluctant to make significant but necessary changes after so much investment. One way of getting some self-objectivity is to put 'some distance' between us and the work. We can do this by leaving the piece for a day or two. This allows us to return to it with fresh eyes and we are more likely to look at it objectively. Reading a large body of work aloud from hard copy forces us to slow down and actually look at the words. This avoids the temptation to skim read and so miss errors, poor expressions, faulty grammar and so on.

The key to reviewing one's own work is to be ruthless. This approach is helpful in getting rid of unnecessary 'filler' words, expressions and general clutter. We have looked at this concept already in Chapter Three when creating written information for clinical trial subjects. Another potential source of clutter is the overuse of clichés. A good definition of a cliché is a 'worn out expression'. Filling our prose with them can give it a tired feel, literally. Many are unnecessary, often don't make sense and add no value to the work. Perhaps worse, they diminish the impact of what it is we are trying to say. Sometimes clichés can be useful to make a point but they should be used sparingly. Here are a few examples. You can probably think of your own favourite toe-curlers to add to this list.

The Institute of Clinical Research

It goes without saying
The proof of the pudding
Having said that
Interesting to note
Well-trodden path
Sadly lacking
Marked contrast
Bitter disappointment
Slowly but surely
Last but not least
Food for thought
Few and far between
Right across the board
Bring to the table
Moving/going forwards
A raft of measures
Take on board
Against a backdrop of...
Explore every avenue
Low/high profile
In the pipeline
To all intents and purposes
In all honesty
An unbroken string of
A vexed question
Cheek by jowl
Caught between two stools
Caught between a rock and a hard place
This is not rocket science
A moot point
Heads up
It's a big ask

Part of the review process involves looking for mistakes in punctuation and grammar. If you are not sure of the rules there are plenty of helpful books on the subject. Some common mistakes in grammar involve the use of apostrophes. 'The student's books' means the books of one student. 'The students' books' refers to the books of two or more students. There is often confusion about the use of 'its' and 'it's'. "It's is a shortened version of 'it is'. 'Its' is known as a 'determiner' and is used to mean 'belonging to' or 'associated with'. For example we might be writing about the books in a library. 'Its books' refers to the books of the library.

Reviewing is best done in one sitting if possible. If the volume of work is very large then a concentrated effort over a few days is necessary. Finding a quiet place where you will be undisturbed is ideal. This allows you to sustain a continuous train of thought and process. You are more likely to be consistent in your review doing it this way.

If you are proofreading a final draft of work received from a printer, there are standard symbols which can be used to highlight where changes need to be made. These let the printer know what you would like altered. There are various standards which can be used, one of which is British Standard BS 5261. If you don't do proofreading for publication regularly then you can put a circle around the text that needs to be altered and write instructions in the margin explaining what needs to be done.

Reviewing other people's work

When we are reviewing other people's work we need to be clear about our purpose. Are we being asked to proofread something? In that case we need to use the same techniques as we have in reviewing our own. If we are reviewing work to pass judgement on a report or technical/scientific information (as a peer reviewer for example), then we must assume the proof reading has been done. Our role here is to evaluate the reasoning, arguments put forward, assumptions made and check facts for soundness.

The major difference between reviewing our own work and other people's is that we need to give him/her our comments and feedback. If we are looking over a piece of work from a relatively junior member of staff (for example a report), they may not have much if any experience of writing. We will look for the obvious aspects like correct use of English, clarity of meaning and so on. We want the content to be correct. The danger in being over-critical is that we alter the style to suit our own. This can have the effect of reducing the impact of a document and breaking up its rhythm. Marking text with large amounts of unnecessary petty changes or corrections can be detrimental and undermine the confidence of an inexperienced writer. An important aspect is to make this a valuable learning experience. Rather than returning a document covered in red comments and corrections, a better way is to do this face-to-face. This gives our trainee writer the chance to appraise their own work and explain why they might have taken a particular approach used a certain expression, etc. Talking face-to-face also helps us to give feedback in the context in which we intended it. Feedback should be specific and cover positive aspects of the work and areas for improvement. It should concentrate on the important features of the document. Is the structure of the piece logical and can the reader navigate it easily? Check that points are adequately made and followed up with the right amount of explanation. Look for anything that is obviously missing or in the wrong place.

Reviewing a non-native English speaker's piece of work should be done with tact and sensitivity. English as a foreign language can be difficult to master. There are so many words to choose from (English is said to have more words than any other language) and some words with the same spelling have several meanings. Some examples of words with similar spellings and different meanings include these.

• Affect(v) = to produce an effect on or to pretend • Effect (v) = to bring about or to accomplish
• Altogether = entirely, totally • All together = all at the same time
• Compliment = an expression of praise • Complement = that which makes something complete
• Credible = convincing • Creditable = deserving praise
• Dependant (n) = one who depends on another • Dependent (adj) = depending, needing the help of
• Ensure = to make safe or certain • Assure = to declare, to promise • Insure = to protect (by contract of insurance)
• Personal = one's own • Personnel = body of people employed at work
• Principle (n) = a basic truth or law • Principal (adj) = chief or leading
• Stationary (adj) = at rest, motionless • Stationery (n) = writing paper etc.
• Lose (v) = to mislay, to be deprived of • Loose (adj) = freed from bonds, not fixed
• Passed = to have been transferred, to have gone etc. • Past = time gone by
• Breath = (n) the air inhaled or exhaled during breathing • Breathe (v) = to take in and exhale air
• Imply = to hint • Infer = to reach an opinion, to reason
• Partially (adv) = to a limited extent (eg partially sighted) • Partly = as regards one part (eg the study is conducted partly in Europe)
• Practice (n) = action as opposed to theory • Practise (v) = to do something repeatedly in order to become skilful
• Suit (v) = to satisfy, to meet the needs of • Suite (n) = a set of something (e.g. rooms)

Giving feedback should be done objectively, constructively and with diplomacy, when peer reviewing. Feedback should be specific. General or vague statements are frustrating and unhelpful for the writer. 'More emphasis could have been placed on organisational issues and external factors' is a more helpful comment than 'The report was not comprehensive enough in some areas'.

Reviewing written work should be a constructive activity. Feedback should be given in a positive way. The aim is to improve the standard of the work. For less experienced members of staff this can be a valuable learning experience in improving their writing skills without inhibiting their natural style.

Chapter Seven: Getting published

Why bother?

Getting your work published can be a really rewarding experience. Seeing one's own name in print for the first time can be a proud moment. The feeling of creating a unique piece of work can bring a great sense of achievement.

From a practical point of view, getting your name in print can get you noticed. This may be very good for business if you are a freelancer particularly if you are trying to make your name in a niche market. You can demonstrate the breadth and depth of your knowledge of your specialist area in a well-drafted piece of work. You may even, over time, establish yourself as a 'guru' in your field. On the other hand, if you work for a company or organisation there may some new business generated as a result of your penmanship. Your career prospects will not be harmed if this happens.

Another consequence of having work published may be an invitation to speak at a seminar or conference. Organisers of these events will often scan journals for potential speakers, especially if they have a particular slot to fill for example 'Electronic Data Capture from a Study Coordinator's Perspective. 'Alternatively you may be invited to sit on expert working parties or committees.

Aside from the potential career and business gains, writing to publish can contribute to personal development. Before putting pen to paper a certain degree of research is usually necessary leading to the inevitable increase in your knowledge of the subject matter.

Making a start

If you are thinking of taking writing seriously and want to get published it is not as difficult as you may think. Writing articles for magazines or journals is an excellent way to start for a number of reasons. The good news is that many clinical research, regulatory and pharmaceutical journals (including Clinical Research focus!) are often looking for articles. Most articles are relatively short, being anything from 1500 to 3000 words long. So if you are undecided about whether writing is for you in the long term, you can find out using only a moderate amount of effort and energy. If you are taking writing more seriously, perhaps with a book in mind, article writing is a good way of learning about developing your style, working to deadlines, structuring your work, and so on. Getting published in a journal may lead to offers of a greater body of work such as writing a chapter for a book or even a complete volume.

One of the toughest aspects of writing on a large scale is finding the time to do it. Most organisations will expect you to do this in your own time outside work. It is also worth noting that if you write in your work time, the piece of work often becomes the property of the company in which you are employed,

The Institute of Clinical Research

even if you are writing it without your employer's knowledge, or even in the field of your work. It's worth being careful in considering this prior to accepting an offer to write an article or a book. The publisher may also wish to retain copyright, and it's important to mention this to your employer if you decide to write during working hours. Any agreements that you sign with the publisher, should be looked over by your company's legal secretary, to ensure that all issues relating to copyright have been agreed by all parties.

Working from home or from the office requires good discipline and it can be useful to break the work down into short concentrated sessions, which will allow you to make surprisingly good progress. Working one hour a day you can make reasonable headway.

Each journal will have its own target readership so every issue will need to appeal to these important customers. Before deciding to write for a particular publication, it is a good idea to read several back issues to get a flavour of the content, the subjects covered, the length of the articles the level of detail, formality of style and the journal's general approach. Many publishers also give authors a writer's guide containing the journal's style and the editor's expectation from your article. By reading this before writing your article, you are closer to getting published.

Arranging your material

Once you have decided on the journal you want to write for and the scope of your article, the next step is to prepare your material. The first step is to create the content. A blank page can be quiet intimidating so a technique known as mind mapping may solve this problem. Originated in the late 1960s by Tony Buzan, a psychologist and mathematician, mind mapping involves using the brain to collect and link related pieces of information.

A mind map is a pictorial representation of a network or cognitive map. Its form can involve images, words, and lines, and can be arranged according to the spatial arrangement of concepts in the mind. The ideas can be organised into groups, branches, or areas. As an example, we may have decided to write an article about how audits and regulatory inspections are conducted. Our mind map might start off looking like this.

Figure 2 Mindmap

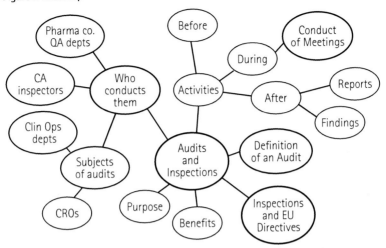

One idea can quickly lead to another and very soon it is possible to compile enough topics for an article. The next stage is to select the topics. We need to decide what is essential to include, the 'must haves'; what we should include if possible and what would be nice to include if there was room. Because journal articles have word limits, we must make sure we include all the essentials while sacrificing some or most of the 'nice to haves'. We may have to lose some of the 'shoulds' as well.

Now we need to put our topics in a logical order so that the reader can make sense of where the piece of work is going. With a topic like auditing, a 'before, during and after' structure is probably the obvious one to go for. Other possibilities may be 'past, present and future' or 'situation, problems, solutions, result'. To create the detail we may need to do some research which might need to be referenced. We may have to consult subject matter experts and these people will need to be acknowledged at the end of the article. Many people find collecting the information and writing the body of the text fairly straightforward. The difficulty comes in making the article interesting for the reader and getting it off to a good start and finish.

Beginnings and endings

Let's deal with the start first. The most important part of any article is the opening paragraph. If you do not capture your reader's interest at this stage there is little chance that they will continue reading after the first few lines. One way to do this is to get the reader to use their imagination. You can do this by asking a question or getting the reader to think about finding themselves in a particular situation. Supposing you had been asked to write an article on the history of GCP, a potentially dry subject. You might try something like this:

'Imagine that you woke up one morning with a raging temperature and blinding headache. You would probably struggle to your medicine cabinet and take some aspirin or paracetamol or both. Now picture the same situation, but instead, it is two hundred years ago. How would you be able to treat yourself then, if at all?'

You could continue by introducing the idea of having some medicine you could trust and rely on. Then bring in the concepts of establishing efficacy and safety by clinical research carried out within a framework of GCP and you're away!

Another technique is to start with a mystery. Here is an example:

'Last year a remarkable exhibit came to light. Hidden in the vaults of a London museum was a scrap of paper containing a few strands of hair. The paper was crudely fashioned into an envelope but the words on it immediately caused a stir: Hair of His Late Majesty, King George 3rd.'

Analysis of the hair showed that it was laden with vast levels of arsenic. It contained over 300 times the toxic level. Scientists were baffled at how such large amounts of such a hazardous compound came to be there. Further research revealed that arsenic was one of the compounds used to treat porphyria, the bizarre and debilitating condition from which the King suffered.

Now you can continue with something about how nowadays a member of the royal family (or anyone else) could not be treated by the medical profession in such a fog of ignorance because of the advent of an ethical and systematic approach to drug development.

A third method is to make a surprising statement or perhaps something that will shock but not in a sensational way. Here is a sample of one.

'In 1997 President Clinton made the following apology to the remaining eight survivors of one of the worst scandals in clinical research of the 20th century. "The United States government did something that was wrong- deeply, profoundly, morally wrong. It was an outrage to our commitment to integrity and equality for all our citizens"

The language President Clinton uses is understandably emotive. It opens the door for you to expand upon this tragedy, the Tuskegee Syphilis Study, – as an example of unethical clinical research. This can lead onto how ethical issues have moulded the regulations. Then you can bring in other aspects such as events caused more by ignorance than intent. Examples include the thalidomide and sulphanilamide tragedies of the 20th century.

Closing a piece of working can sometimes be harder than starting. We need to try and leave the reader with a lasting impression. Bringing the article to close too abruptly or letting it drift towards no obvious conclusion is not very rewarding for us or our audience. We need a powerful close to leave our reader with a memorable image.

There are various methods that are worth trying. The first is to pose a question perhaps about where the future may lead. Returning to our article on the history of GCP it might look something like this.

'We have seen the past and how tragedies and human rights abuses have often been the trigger for new GCP legislation. What new challenges will clinical research bring as we face more complex choices in the treatment of disease and as we venture into new geographical territories?'

A second method is to issue a challenge, perhaps something a little controversial?

'New technology and electronic data capture in particular are changing our industry forever. The days of the CRA as merely a detector and a corrector of errors are over. We need to adopt a preventative approach to raising standards of GCP. Only then will we be able to face the increasingly complicated and competitive field of drug development.'

The danger is of over sensationalising, so some judgement is needed. Lastly we can present our theme in a wider context.

'So far a coordinated approach to GCP has been taken between the USA, Japan and the European Union. Clinical research is becoming increasingly global and is being conducted on an ever-growing section of the world's population. The days of GCH GCP, a Global Conference on Harmonisation cannot be too far away.'

Maintaining interest

It will be a shame if we have worked hard at creating a bright opening only to bore the reader soon afterwards with a series of turgid fact laden passages. If we have got rid of unnecessary words, expressions, and tired clichés we will already have gone a long way to sharpening up our text and giving it some vibrancy and punch. What are some of the other techniques we can use?

Try thinking about your favourite books. What was it that meant you 'couldn't put it down'? What did the writer do to make you so eager to find out what was going to happen next?

A good novelist can paint mental pictures for us so well, that we can imagine being there with the characters in the book. The same methods can be used for scientific and factual pieces of work. One of the most successful scientific books has been Stephen Hawking's 'Brief History of Time'. The book has been translated into 40 languages and has sold over nine million copies. It tackles the potentially baffling subjects of cosmology, quantum physics and Einstein's General Theory of Relativity. Hawking's straightforward and simple style with the clever use of metaphors and analogies has given us a fascinating insight into the forces that shape our universe.

A metaphor is a figure of speech applied to an object or person that it does not literally stand for. The idea is to imply a resemblance. Original metaphors can be quite effective and can liven up a piece of writing. Worn out ones have become clichés. 'The European Clinical Trial Directive has produced a minefield of legislation.' is an example of one. This metaphor sets a rather negative tone, either intentionally or otherwise. The use of the word "minefield" implies a complicated hazard where great care is needed not to come to harm. Another attempt, with a musical theme might go something like this. 'The European Commission has tried to harmonise clinical research in the EU by orchestrating the European Clinical Trial Directive.' Using the word 'orchestrating' reinforces the concept of harmony and coordination.

Analogies are less subtle than metaphors. An analogy is a comparison designed to explain a concept or idea by showing similarity. 'An atom is like a mini solar system' is an example of one. The comparison does not have to be strictly true. The aim is to give the reader a reference point of familiarity so that they get a general picture. Avoid using analogies inappropriately with comparisons which may mean nothing to some of the readers. Saying 'Trying to keep clinical trial projects to their original timelines is like a car journey on the M25, you can guarantee delays', is not a particularly useful analogy to someone who is not British and who may not be familiar with the frequent hold-ups on this motorway. 'Managing a clinical trial project without measuring progress is like climbing Everest blindfolded' has universal understanding. Everyone has heard about the perils of climbing Mount Everest and we can all imagine what it is like to be blindfolded.

Writing a book

If you develop a taste for writing by contributing articles to journals you may want to try something more ambitious, like a book. Finding something to write about which is both factual and original is tough. There are numerous volumes about clinical research in print. However you might have a particular interest or angle which is covered relatively sparsely. Something like 'Conducting Clinical Trials in Developing Countries' might be a subject which you may know much about already and which you feel there is a demand for. Trying to identify a gap in the market is very important. If you want to get into print you are going to have to convince at least one publisher that your book is a worthwhile project. If you are a first-time author you will need to write the manuscript first and then find a publisher. At the very least, you will need to have your outline, or synopsis, prepared with a few sample chapters to present to the publisher. Many publishers may want some input into the content of the book, in particular in scientific writing. Very few companies will take a chance with an unknown author without seeing their work first. However, it is possible to meet publishers at various events, such as conferences, to discuss your idea and then possibly taking it further. Not many people start and finish writing a book, so if you do achieve it you will become a member of a pretty exclusive club. The financial rewards for most works of non-fiction are not great, so your motivation will probably come from the satisfaction of having created something unique and perhaps opening a new perspective on clinical research.

Planning a book is like preparing to write an article but on a grander scale. Most books tend to be in the order of 50000 to 120000 words. Your first task is to rough out the scope of what your book will cover and how many words approximately it will contain. Then decide on the chapter headings. At this stage write a synopsis of your book. This should be about 100 - 200 words. The synopsis is useful in keeping you on track and you will need it for publishers, literary agents or professional reviewers. Prepare the outlines of each chapter using the techniques we have discussed earlier such as mind mapping. This will give you the 'must haves', 'should haves' and 'nice to haves' for each chapter. A working title for your book is helpful at this stage. Once you have finished writing the manuscript, a better title may occur to you or you may decide to stick with the original one. The publisher may also suggest a title for your piece of work.

You will probably need to research your content. Articles from journals, information from other books and the Internet are all useful starting points. Make sure your sources are reliable and that you acknowledge them. If you find you are building up a lengthy list of references some bibliographic software may be worth investing in. Bibliographic software packages are specialised databases. They are designed to create a bibliography from the references that you quote. The software provides support for reference formats and gives you the ability to generate specific bibliographic formats. They are particularly useful as you can populate the database with references from the start, and not leave it to the last minute, which often means you have to find the references that you have forgot to acknowledge.

Because writing a book can be a lengthy project it is important to keep the momentum going. Writing something little and often is better than leaving the work for long periods and trying to produce large blocks in intense bursts. A steady stream of effort helps with continuity, cross-referencing between chapters, and avoids accidental omissions, repetition and disjointed work. Five hundred words a day is achievable and averages out to about 90 minutes of effort. If you can plug away at this rate then you should have a manuscript ready for review and editing after about 4 - 6 months.

Review your work ruthlessly for clutter, sense, style, sentence and paragraph structure. Polish the text, strive for consistency and check the formatting. Make sure you reference as you go along. Ensure you number the pages. This is particularly important when you come to print the manuscript. Dropping the printed work and watching it scatter across the floor is bad enough. Trying to put it back together in the right order without page numbers is like trying to do one of those jigsaw puzzles where half the pieces are an identical shade of sky blue.

The Institute of Clinical Research

Finding a publisher

This is the hardest stage of getting a book into print. Publishers get hundreds of manuscripts to look at and reject the great majority of them. The first step is to find publishers who specialise in scientific non-fiction. Most publishers have guidelines for authors. These include specifications for font size, line spacing, length in words of the manuscript and synopsis. Some publishers might ask you for a brief biography and in some cases an administration fee.

When sending a manuscript make sure it is to the publisher's specifications. A fancy font on exotic coloured paper will get your work noticed but not for the right reasons. There is no need to put your work in a binder or staple it together. Loose leaf in an envelope will be enough to keep your numbered pages together. The synopsis should be at the top. This is what the publisher will read first before deciding to go any further. Write a brief covering letter. If you want your manuscript returned, enclose a stamped addressed envelope.

Most manuscripts get a rejection slip. You can increase your chances of success by sending your work to companies offering professional critiquing services. For a fee they will read your entire manuscript and give you feedback on how to make it more publishable. If they like your work they may introduce you to literary agents or publishers as part of the service.

Getting published is hard going. But like anything which is tough, if you persevere and are prepared to listen to, accept, and act on criticism, it is very rewarding when you succeed.

The Institute of Clinical Research

Conclusion

We all write something most days at work. We have looked at the range of uses writing skills can be put to by the clinical research professional. We have seen how one of the most important aspects is putting ourselves in the shoes of the reader. Thinking about the result of what we want to achieve by our writing is also important. Clarity and brevity are key factors in delivering the message. These aspects are sometimes hard to achieve, given the rich nature of the English language.

Sometimes writing is not the most appropriate form of communication. Part of the skill of a writer is knowing when to use other media to deliver the message especially if it is bad news or a sensitive issue. Its use in clinical research is particularly important in creating and maintaining a robust audit trail that can be consulted years after the trial's completion. A written piece of work should always be created with an end purpose in mind. As F. Scott Fitzgerald once said: "The reason one writes isn't the fact he wants to say something. He writes because he has something to say."

The Institute of Clinical Research

References

International Conference on Harmonisation of Technical Requirements for Registration of Pharmaceuticals for Human Use (ICH) Harmonised Tripartite Guideline for Good Clinical Practice (GCP), 1 May 1996

Phythian, B.A., Correct English, Hodder and Stoughton, 1992